THE CASTOR OIL BIBLE PROGRAM

Simple and easy solution to caster oil, more than 100+ recipes of castor oil to bring your natural beauty and healthy to your table.

JENNIFER .S COLE

TABLE OF CONTENT

INTRODUCTION

Introducing the Castor Oil Bible Program: Your Comprehensive Guide to Harnessing the Power of Nature's Miracle Elixir!

Welcome to a journey of discovery, healing, and transformation with the Castor Oil Bible Program. In this groundbreaking program, we delve into the incredible world of castor oil—a time-honored remedy cherished for its remarkable healing properties and boundless potential.

Are you ready to unlock the secrets of this ancient elixir and revolutionize your approach to health and wellness? Look no further than the Castor Oil Bible Program, your trusted companion on the path to vibrant living.

Join us as we explore the rich history and fascinating origins of castor oil, tracing its roots back through centuries of traditional medicine and folk remedies. Learn how this versatile oil is extracted and produced, and gain a deeper understanding of its chemical composition and therapeutic benefits.

But that's just the beginning. With the Castor Oil Bible Program, you'll discover a treasure trove of practical tips, expert advice, and innovative recipes for incorporating castor oil into every aspect of your life. From soothing skincare treatments to invigorating hair masks, from digestive health remedies to immune-boosting elixirs—our comprehensive guide covers it all.

But the Castor Oil Bible Program is more than just a book—it's a transformative experience designed to empower you on your journey to optimal health and well-being. With our step-by-step instructions, easy-to-follow recipes, and expert guidance, you'll learn how to harness the full potential of castor oil and embrace a natural, holistic approach to self-care.

Are you ready to embark on a journey of wellness and vitality? Join us in the Castor Oil Bible Program and discover the extraordinary benefits of nature's miracle elixir. Let's unlock the power of castor oil together and embrace a life of health, beauty, and vitality like never before. Welcome to the Castor Oil Bible Program—where your journey to holistic living begins!

Chapter 1:WHAT EXACTLY IS CASTOR OIL:

Vegetable oil called castor oil is extracted from the seeds of the Ricinus communis plant, which produces castor beans. It has been used for medical purposes and in a variety of businesses for a very long time. Key details regarding castor oil are as follows:

Formulation and Removal

About 90% of castor oil is composed of ricinoleic acid, a fatty acid type that is abundant in the oil. Other fatty acids like oleic and linoleic acids are also present.

Extraction: Pressing the castor seeds yields the oil. Solvents or mechanical means can be used for this process.
Applications

Pharmaceutical:

Laxative: Castor oil is widely known for its laxative properties. It causes the intestines to move more, which induces bowel movements.
Labor Induction: This controversial procedure should only be carried out under medical supervision. It is occasionally used to induce labor.
Skin and Hair Care: Because of its moisturizing qualities, it is frequently utilized in cosmetics and hair products. It can aid in the treatment of dry skin and dandruff.

Industrial:

Because of its high viscosity and lubricating qualities, lubricant is used in the production process.

An ingredient used to produce biodiesel is biodiesel.

Plasticizer: A substance used in the making of resins and plastics.

Cosmetic:

Skin Care: Because of its emollient qualities, it can be found in lotions, creams, and soaps.

Hair care: Including hair treatments that encourage healthy scalps and hair development.

Health Advantages and Safety Measures

Anti-inflammatory: When applied topically, castor oil's anti-inflammatory qualities can aid in the treatment of ailments like arthritis and sore muscles.

antibacterial: Its antibacterial qualities can aid in the healing of small cuts and skin infections.

Precautions: Although castor oil has many advantages, it should be used carefully. When taken orally in excessive amounts, it might have adverse effects such as nausea, dehydration, and cramping in the abdomen. When using it to induce labor, pregnant women should speak with a healthcare professional beforehand.

In summary

Castor oil is a multipurpose oil used in cosmetics, manufacturing, and medicine. Its main constituent, ricinoleic acid, gives it special qualities that make it useful for a variety of applications. However, in order to prevent any negative consequences, it should be used carefully.

Chapter 2:ORIGINS AND HISTORY

The Origins and History of Castor Oil

Old Use

Egypt: Castor oil was first used in recorded history in ancient Egypt. Its slow burning characteristic led to its employment as fuel in lamps by the Egyptians, according to archeological discoveries. It was also used as a laxative, in cosmetics, and in medicine. It is said that Cleopatra used castor oil to make her eyes more radiant.

India: Due to its therapeutic qualities, castor oil has been utilized in Ayurvedic medicine there for thousands of years. It was used to cure a wide range of illnesses, such as inflammation, skin disorders, and digestive problems.

Ancient Classics

Greece and Rome: Castor oil was also known to the Greeks and Romans. Its application in medicine was reported by Greek doctors like Hippocrates. The

Romans also employed it, especially as a purgative and for skin treatment.

Medieval Times

Europe: Castor oil was brought to Europe throughout the Middle Ages, and it was mostly utilized there for medicinal purposes even after that. Because of its healing qualities, it was frequently referred to as "Palma Christi" or "Palm of Christ".

Contemporary Period

Industrial Revolution: Castor oil's uses greatly increased when the Industrial Revolution got underway. It was used in machinery for the manufacturing of soaps, dyes, and other compounds due to its lubricating qualities.

20th century: Castor oil was used in the aviation sector to lubricate airplane engines during World Wars I and II.

Manufacturing and Worldwide Distribution

Native Areas: The castor plant, or Ricinus communis, is indigenous to Eastern Africa,

India, and the Southeast Mediterranean Basin. Castor oil is still mostly produced in India, with Brazil and China following closely behind.

Colonialism: The introduction of castor oil manufacturing to various regions of the world was facilitated by European colonization. To satisfy the demand in Europe, the British in especially planted it in their colonies in Africa and India.

Use in Medicine and Cosmetics

19th Century Medicine: Castor oil was widely used as a home treatment during this time, especially in Europe and the United States. It was widely used to treat a wide range of illnesses and as a laxative.

Cosmetic Industry: Due to castor oil's moisturizing qualities, the cosmetic industry started using it in goods in the 20th century. It's still a mainstay in a lot of skincare and hair care products today.

Health & Well-being: Castor oil is utilized in both conventional and alternative medicine nowadays due to its widespread recognition of its health advantages. It can be used to promote hair growth, improve skin health, and cure minor skin infections and inflammations.

Sustainable Industry: Due to its adaptability and ongoing significance in contemporary industry, castor oil is also garnering attention as a sustainable resource in the manufacturing of biodiesel and biodegradable plastics.

The extensive and diverse history of castor oil highlights its significance in many cultures and historical periods, underscoring its versatility and continuing worth.

Chapter 3:EXTRACTION AND PRODUCTION

Castor oil extraction and production

Developing Castor Plants

Climate and Soil: Tropical and subtropical areas are ideal for the growth of castor plants (Ricinus communis). They like warm weather and well-drained soil.

Planting: Usually, seeds are sown right there in the field. In temperate regions, they can grow as annuals, but in tropical areas, they can thrive as perennials.

Growth and Harvest: The plants mature in 140–180 days, growing quickly. Once the seed pods have dried and gone brown, the castor seeds, also known as beans, are harvested.

Procedure for Extraction

Gathering and Preparing Seeds:

The harvested seed pods are gathered and given time to desiccate.

After being taken out of the pods, the seeds are cleaned to get rid of any dirt, debris, or other contaminants.

Applying pressure:

Cold pressing: To extract oil without using heat, seeds are crushed and pressed. Because the oil's natural qualities are preserved, it can be used for both medical and cosmetic purposes.

Hot pressing: Before pressing, seeds are heated, which boosts output but may change some of the characteristics of the oil.

Extracting Solvents:

The residual oil in the pressed seed cake can be extracted in an industrial setting using a solvent like hexane. Afterwards, the solvent evaporates, leaving just pure castor oil remained.

While maximal extraction efficiency is guaranteed by this procedure, solvent residues may need to be removed by additional refining.

Refinement:

To get rid of contaminants, increase stability, and improve clarity, the extracted oil may go through refining.
Degumming, neutralization, bleaching, and deodorization are typical refining procedures.
Hydrogenation: a choice

Castor oil can be hydrogenated to create hydrogenated castor oil (HCO) or castor wax for use in certain industrial applications. By adding hydrogen to the oil under carefully monitored conditions, this procedure modifies the oil's physical characteristics and solidifies it at room temperature.

Manufacturing and International Markets

Top Producers: India produces the most castor oil, accounting for more than 80% of global production. Chinese and Brazilian producers are also noteworthy.

Worldwide Demand: A wide range of industries, including biodiesel, lubricants, cosmetics, and medicines, have a need for castor oil. Its numerous applications keep pushing up output.

Control of Quality

Standards: A number of national and international standards govern the quality of castor oil, guaranteeing uniformity and safety for a range of applications. Testing is frequently done on parameters like acidity, moisture content, and purity.

Certifications: In order to target particular market segments, especially in the food, cosmetic, and pharmaceutical industries, producers may pursue certifications like organic or non-GMO.

The effects on the environment and economy

Sustainability: Because castor oil has a minimal environmental impact, it is regarded as a sustainable crop. The castor plant may thrive on marginal ground unsuitable for food crops because it is resilient and resistant to drought.

Economic Importance: Castor farming is a key source of revenue for smallholder farmers in places like India. The crop is a desirable choice for agricultural growth due to its adaptability and very cheap input requirements.

In summary

To optimize yield and preserve quality, castor oil is produced using a blend of conventional and contemporary methods. Its many uses and adaptability make it a significant commodity in many industries, and its sustainable farming methods add to its expanding worldwide significance.

Chapter 4:CHEMICAL COMPOSITION

The chemical makeup of castor oil

The distinctive qualities and extensive range of applications of castor oil are attributed to its elevated concentration of ricinoleic acid. This is a thorough analysis of its chemical makeup:

Triglycerides make up the majority of castor oil's composition, with the following fatty acids being its most important constituents:

Acid Ricinoleic (C18:1 OH)

85–90% of the total

Properties: Ricinoleic acid is a highly polar and viscous omega-9 fatty acid with a hydroxyl group on its 12th carbon. Castor oil's distinct qualities, including its higher viscosity and high alcohol solubility, are attributed to this hydroxyl group.

C18:1 Oleic Acid

4-6% as a percentage

Oleic acid, an omega-9 fatty acid, adds to the oil's stability and moisturizing qualities.
Acid Linoleic (C18:2)

3-5% as a percentage
Properties: Linoleic acid, an omega-6 fatty acid, is vital to human health and helps maintain hydrated and healthy skin.
Acid Palmitic (C16:0)

1-2% as a percentage
Properties: Palmitic acid, a saturated fatty acid, improves the smoothness and stability of the oil.
Acid Stearic (C18:0)

1-2% as a percentage
Properties: Stearic acid, another saturated fatty acid, improves the creamy texture and moisturizing qualities of the oil.
C18:0 OH, or dihydroxystearic acid

Ratio: Trace elements

Characteristics: Produced by hydrogenating ricinoleic acid, it enhances the stability and viscosity of hydrogenated castor oil.

Smaller Parts

Natural antioxidants called tocopherols, or vitamin E, aid in stabilizing the oil and extending its shelf life.

Plant sterols known as phytosterols are responsible for the anti-inflammatory and skin-soothing effects of the oil.

Properties, both chemical and physical

Viscosity: The high concentration of ricinoleic acid in castor oil makes it noticeably more viscous than other vegetable oils.

Its solubility—it dissolves in alcohol but not in water—allows for a variety of industrial and medicinal uses.

Approximately 313°C (595°F) is the boiling point.

Density: At 20°C, it varies between 0.957 and 0.961 g/cm^3.

Practical attributes

Emollient: The oil is a great moisturizer and skin conditioner due to its high ricinoleic acid concentration.

Humectant: It is useful in skincare and cosmetic formulations because it aids in the retention of moisture.

Lubricant: It is perfect for use in hydraulic fluids and lubricants due to its viscosity and film-forming qualities.

Antimicrobial and Anti-inflammatory: Ricinoleic acid's presence aids in the plant's capacity to lower inflammation and stop the growth of some bacteria and fungi.

Pharmaceutical and Industrial Uses

Cosmetics: Because of its emollient and moisturizing qualities, it is used in skin creams, lotions, and lipsticks.

Pharmaceuticals: Used as a laxative, in topical ointments, and as a drug carrier oil.

Applications in Industry: Used in the manufacture of paints, coatings, lubricants, hydraulic fluids, and biodiesel.

Food Additive: Licensed for use in food as a mold inhibitor and as part of materials used in packaging intended for food usage.

In summary

Because of its distinct qualities that make it desirable in a variety of sectors, castor oil is mostly composed of ricinoleic acid. Its fatty acid composition and smaller constituents support its use as a bio-based industrial material, lubricant, and emollient.

Chapter 5: IMPORTANCE AND USES OF CASTOR OIL

The Value and Applications of Castor Oil

Due to its distinct chemical makeup, especially its high ricinoleic acid content, castor oil has many advantageous qualities that make it useful in a wide range of sectors. Detailed analysis of its significance and applications follows:

Laxative:

Mechanism: Castor oil is a strong laxative stimulant. After consumption, it is converted by the small intestine into ricinoleic acid, which causes the intestines to contract and cause bowel motions.
Use: Before undergoing medical operations, it is used to empty the intestines and relieve constipation.

Induction of Labor:

Customary Use: Due to possible hazards and adverse consequences, this procedure should only be carried out under medical supervision. Nevertheless, it has been traditionally used to induce childbirth.

Relief from pain and anti-inflammatory:

Application: Castor oil can be applied topically to treat illnesses including arthritis and aching muscles by reducing pain and inflammation.

Skin and Injuries Management:

Properties: It works well to cure small cuts, burns, and wounds because of its moisturizing and antibacterial qualities. It aids in maintaining skin hydration, which encourages healing.

Antimicrobial Substance:

Function: Castor oil is effective in treating infections and as a preservative in some items since it has been demonstrated to suppress the growth of many bacterial and fungal pathogens.

Uses for Cosmetics and Personal Care

Skin Maintenance:

Moisturizer: The skin is kept hydrated and smooth by the emollient qualities of this product.

Anti-aging: Castor oil, which is high in fatty acids, can increase skin elasticity and lessen the visibility of wrinkles.

Hair Maintenance:

Hair Growth: To promote hair growth, lessen hair loss, and enhance scalp health, hair growth treatments frequently contain this ingredient.

Conditioner: A frequent element in conditioners and hair oils, it helps to bring shine and smoothness to hair.

Lip Maintenance:

Lip Balms: Because of its thick consistency and moisturizing qualities, castor oil is a common ingredient in lip balms and glosses.

Cosmetics:

Ingredient: For its smooth application and long-lasting effects, this ingredient is used in many beauty products, such as eyeliners and mascaras.

Industrial Applications

Grease:

Properties: High-performance lubricants and hydraulic fluids can benefit from the high viscosity and lubricity of castor oil.

Biodegradability: Because of its biodegradability, it is a recommended option for applications that are sensitive to the environment.

Biodiesel:

Production: Biodiesel is made from castor oil, which provides a sustainable and renewable fuel supply.

Polymers and Plastics:

Plasticizer: It enhances the flexibility and durability of some plastics by acting as a plasticizer during manufacture.

Polymers: Biodegradable polymers and resins are made from castor oil derivatives.

Paints and Coatings:

Use: Because of its superior drying qualities, it is used in the manufacturing of coatings, paints, and varnishes.

Cleaners and Soaps:

Saponification: Castor oil's moisturizing properties and capacity to generate a

consistent lather make it a useful ingredient in soap production.
Uses in Agriculture
Chemical pesticides:

Natural Pesticide: Castor oil works particularly well against moles and voles as a natural pesticide and insect repellent.
Applying fertilizers:

Source of Nutrients: A byproduct of oil extraction called castor seed cake is utilized as an organic fertilizer that is high in nitrogen and other nutrients.
In summary
The fact that castor oil is so widely used in industry, agriculture, cosmetics, and medicine speaks volumes about its adaptability. Due to its special qualities, which result from its high ricinoleic acid content, it can be used as an essential component in many different goods and applications, underscoring its significance and usefulness on a global scale.

1. Hair Growth Serum

Ingredients:

- 2 tablespoons castor oil
- 1 tablespoon coconut oil
- 1 tablespoon argan oil
- 10 drops rosemary essential oil

Instructions:

1. Combine castor oil, coconut oil, and argan oil in a small bowl.
2. Add rosemary essential oil and mix well.
3. Apply the mixture to your scalp and massage gently for 5-10 minutes.

4. Leave it on for at least 2 hours or overnight for best results.
5. Wash your hair with a mild shampoo and conditioner.
6. Use this treatment 2-3 times a week.

2. Deep Conditioning Hair Mask

Ingredients:

- 2 tablespoons castor oil
- 1 ripe avocado
- 1 tablespoon honey

Instructions:

1. Mash the avocado in a bowl until smooth.
2. Add castor oil and honey to the avocado and mix thoroughly.

3. Apply the mixture to damp hair, focusing on the ends.
4. Cover your hair with a shower cap and leave it on for 30-60 minutes.
5. Rinse thoroughly and shampoo as usual.
6. Use this mask once a week for soft, hydrated hair.

3. Eyelash and Eyebrow Growth Serum

Ingredients:

- 1 tablespoon castor oil
- 1 tablespoon aloe vera gel
- 5 drops vitamin E oil

Instructions:

1. Mix castor oil, aloe vera gel, and vitamin E oil in a small bowl.
2. Transfer the mixture to a clean mascara tube or small container.
3. Apply the serum to your eyelashes and eyebrows using a clean spoolie brush before bed.
4. Leave it on overnight and wash off in the morning.
5. Use nightly for best results.

4. Hydrating Face Serum

Ingredients:

- 1 tablespoon castor oil
- 1 tablespoon jojoba oil
- 5 drops lavender essential oil

Instructions:

1. Combine castor oil and jojoba oil in a small bottle.
2. Add lavender essential oil and shake well to mix.
3. Apply a few drops of the serum to your face and neck after cleansing, massaging gently into the skin.
4. Use this serum nightly for a hydrating boost.

5. Anti-Aging Eye Cream

Ingredients:

- 1 tablespoon castor oil
- 1 tablespoon shea butter
- 5 drops frankincense essential oil

Instructions:

1. Melt the shea butter in a double boiler until it becomes liquid.
2. Remove from heat and mix in castor oil and frankincense essential oil.
3. Pour the mixture into a small container and let it cool and solidify.
4. Gently apply a small amount of the cream around the eye area before bed.
5. Use nightly to help reduce the appearance of fine lines and wrinkles.

6. Nourishing Nail and Cuticle Oil

Ingredients:

- 1 tablespoon castor oil
- 1 tablespoon olive oil
- 5 drops tea tree essential oil

Instructions:

1. Mix castor oil and olive oil in a small bowl.
2. Add tea tree essential oil and stir well.
3. Apply a small amount of the oil to your nails and cuticles, massaging gently.
4. Use this treatment daily to keep nails and cuticles nourished and strong.

7. Soothing Lip Balm

Ingredients:

- 1 tablespoon castor oil
- 1 tablespoon coconut oil
- 1 tablespoon beeswax pellets
- 5 drops peppermint essential oil

Instructions:

1. Melt the beeswax pellets and coconut oil in a double boiler until fully melted.
2. Remove from heat and stir in castor oil and peppermint essential oil.
3. Pour the mixture into small lip balm containers or tubes and let it cool and solidify.
4. Apply to your lips as needed for hydration and soothing relief.

1. Castor Oil Detox Drink

Ingredients:

- 1 teaspoon castor oil (food grade)
- 1 cup warm water
- 1 tablespoon lemon juice
- 1 teaspoon honey (optional)

Instructions:

1. Warm the water to a comfortable drinking temperature.
2. Add the castor oil, lemon juice, and honey (if using).
3. Stir well until all ingredients are combined.
4. Drink this mixture on an empty stomach once a week to help cleanse your digestive system.

2. Ginger and Castor Oil Tea

Ingredients:

- 1 teaspoon castor oil (food grade)
- 1 cup water
- 1 teaspoon grated fresh ginger
- 1 tablespoon lemon juice
- 1 teaspoon honey (optional)

Instructions:

1. Boil the water and add the grated ginger.
2. Let it simmer for 5-10 minutes, then strain the tea into a cup.
3. Add the castor oil, lemon juice, and honey (if using).
4. Stir well and drink this tea once or twice a week to aid digestion and reduce bloating.

3. Castor Oil and Apple Cider Vinegar Drink

Ingredients:

- 1 teaspoon castor oil (food grade)
- 1 tablespoon apple cider vinegar
- 1 cup warm water
- 1 teaspoon honey (optional)

Instructions:

1. Warm the water and pour it into a cup.
2. Add the castor oil, apple cider vinegar, and honey (if using).
3. Mix well and drink this concoction in the morning on an empty stomach once or twice a week.

4. Herbal Castor Oil Smoothie

Ingredients:

- 1 teaspoon castor oil (food grade)
- 1 cup unsweetened almond milk
- 1 cup spinach leaves
- 1/2 cucumber, chopped
- 1 green apple, cored and chopped
- 1 tablespoon chia seeds

Instructions:

1. Combine all ingredients in a blender.
2. Blend until smooth.
3. Drink this smoothie as a breakfast replacement once a week for a nutrient-packed detoxifying meal.

5. Castor Oil and Turmeric Detox Shot

Ingredients:

- 1/2 teaspoon castor oil (food grade)
- 1/2 teaspoon ground turmeric
- 1 tablespoon lemon juice
- 1/2 cup warm water
- Pinch of black pepper

Instructions:

1. Warm the water and pour it into a small cup.
2. Add the castor oil, turmeric, lemon juice, and black pepper.
3. Stir well and drink this detox shot in the morning on an empty stomach once a week.

6. Cleansing Green Juice with Castor Oil

Ingredients:

- 1 teaspoon castor oil (food grade)
- 1 cucumber
- 1 celery stalk
- 1 handful of parsley
- 1 green apple, cored and chopped
- 1/2 lemon, juiced

Instructions:

1. Juice the cucumber, celery, parsley, and green apple.
2. Add the lemon juice and castor oil to the green juice.
3. Stir well and drink this juice as a morning cleanser once or twice a week.

7. **Castor Oil and Aloe Vera Detox Drink**

Ingredients:

- 1 teaspoon castor oil (food grade)
- 1/2 cup pure aloe vera juice
- 1 cup coconut water
- 1 tablespoon lime juice

Instructions:

1. Mix all the ingredients in a glass.
2. Stir well until combined.
3. Drink this detoxifying beverage in the morning on an empty stomach once a week to help maintain digestive health and hydration.

Note:

- Moderation: These recipes incorporate small amounts of castor oil to avoid potential side effects like abdominal cramping or diarrhea. Always use food-grade castor oil and consult with a healthcare provider before starting any new dietary regimen, especially if you have underlying health conditions.
- Balanced Diet: These recipes should complement a balanced diet and regular exercise for effective weight maintenance.

1. Castor Oil Lemon Detox Drink

Ingredients:

- 1 teaspoon castor oil (food grade)
- 1 cup warm water
- 1 tablespoon lemon juice
- 1 teaspoon honey (optional)

Instructions:

1. Warm the water to a comfortable drinking temperature.
2. Add the castor oil, lemon juice, and honey (if using).
3. Stir well until all ingredients are combined.
4. Drink this mixture in the morning on an empty stomach once a week to help

cleanse and stimulate your digestive system.

2. Ginger and Castor Oil Tea

Ingredients:

- 1 teaspoon castor oil (food grade)
- 1 cup water
- 1 teaspoon grated fresh ginger
- 1 tablespoon lemon juice
- 1 teaspoon honey (optional)

Instructions:

1. Boil the water and add the grated ginger.
2. Let it simmer for 5-10 minutes, then strain the tea into a cup.

3. Add the castor oil, lemon juice, and honey (if using).
4. Stir well and drink this tea once or twice a week to aid digestion and reduce bloating.

3. **Castor Oil and Apple Cider Vinegar Drink**

Ingredients:

- 1 teaspoon castor oil (food grade)
- 1 tablespoon apple cider vinegar
- 1 cup warm water
- 1 teaspoon honey (optional)

Instructions:

1. Warm the water and pour it into a cup.

2. Add the castor oil, apple cider vinegar, and honey (if using).

3. Mix well and drink this concoction in the morning on an empty stomach once or twice a week to support digestive health.

4. Digestive Health Smoothie

Ingredients:

- 1 teaspoon castor oil (food grade)
- 1 cup unsweetened almond milk
- 1 cup spinach leaves
- 1/2 cucumber, chopped
- 1 green apple, cored and chopped
- 1 tablespoon chia seeds

Instructions:

1. Combine all ingredients in a blender.
2. Blend until smooth.
3. Drink this smoothie as a breakfast replacement once a week for a nutrient-packed digestive boost.

5. Castor Oil and Turmeric Shot

Ingredients:

- 1/2 teaspoon castor oil (food grade)
- 1/2 teaspoon ground turmeric
- 1 tablespoon lemon juice
- 1/2 cup warm water
- Pinch of black pepper

Instructions:

1. Warm the water and pour it into a small cup.

2. Add the castor oil, turmeric, lemon juice, and black pepper.
3. Stir well and drink this shot in the morning on an empty stomach once a week to support digestion and reduce inflammation.

6. **Cleansing Green Juice with Castor Oil**

Ingredients:

- 1 teaspoon castor oil (food grade)
- 1 cucumber
- 1 celery stalk
- 1 handful of parsley
- 1 green apple, cored and chopped
- 1/2 lemon, juiced

Instructions:

1. Juice the cucumber, celery, parsley, and green apple.
2. Add the lemon juice and castor oil to the green juice.
3. Stir well and drink this juice in the morning as a digestive cleanser once or twice a week.

7. Castor Oil and Aloe Vera Digestive Drink

Ingredients:

- 1 teaspoon castor oil (food grade)
- 1/2 cup pure aloe vera juice
- 1 cup coconut water
- 1 tablespoon lime juice

Instructions:

1. Mix all the ingredients in a glass.
2. Stir well until combined.
3. Drink this digestive health beverage in the morning on an empty stomach once a week to help maintain digestive health and hydration.

Note:

- Moderation: These recipes incorporate small amounts of castor oil to avoid potential side effects like abdominal cramping or diarrhea. Always use food-grade castor oil and consult with a healthcare provider before starting any new dietary regimen, especially if you have underlying health conditions.
- Balanced Diet: These recipes should complement a balanced diet and regular exercise for effective digestive health maintenance.

1. **Castor Oil Chest Rub**

Ingredients:

- 2 tablespoons castor oil
- 1 tablespoon coconut oil
- 10 drops eucalyptus essential oil
- 10 drops peppermint essential oil

Instructions:

1. Melt the coconut oil if it's solid.
2. Mix the castor oil and coconut oil in a small bowl.
3. Add eucalyptus and peppermint essential oils.
4. Stir well and apply the mixture to your chest and throat.

5. Cover with a warm cloth and relax for 20-30 minutes.
6. Use this rub once a day to relieve congestion and support easier breathing.

2. Castor Oil Steam Inhalation

Ingredients:

- 1 tablespoon castor oil
- 5 drops eucalyptus essential oil
- 5 drops tea tree essential oil
- 1 bowl of hot water

Instructions:

1. Pour hot water into a large bowl.
2. Add castor oil, eucalyptus oil, and tea tree oil to the water.

3. Lean over the bowl, cover your head with a towel, and inhale the steam deeply for 10-15 minutes.
4. Repeat this treatment once a day to clear nasal and chest congestion.

3. Castor Oil and Garlic Chest Pack

Ingredients:

- 2 tablespoons castor oil
- 2 cloves garlic, crushed

Instructions:

1. Warm the castor oil slightly.
2. Add the crushed garlic to the warm castor oil and let it infuse for 10 minutes.
3. Strain out the garlic pieces.

4. Apply the infused oil to your chest and cover with a warm cloth or towel.
5. Leave it on for 20-30 minutes to help with congestion and respiratory discomfort.
6. Use this treatment once a day when experiencing symptoms.

4. Castor Oil and Ginger Compress

Ingredients:

- 2 tablespoons castor oil
- 1 tablespoon grated fresh ginger

Instructions:

1. Warm the castor oil slightly.
2. Add the grated ginger and let it infuse for 10 minutes.

3. Strain out the ginger pieces.
4. Soak a cloth in the warm oil mixture and apply it to your chest.
5. Cover with a dry towel and leave it on for 20-30 minutes.
6. Use this compress once a day to relieve respiratory symptoms.

5. Castor Oil and Turmeric Paste

Ingredients:

- 2 tablespoons castor oil
- 1 teaspoon ground turmeric

Instructions:

1. Mix castor oil and ground turmeric in a small bowl to form a paste.

2. Apply the paste to your chest and throat.
3. Cover with a warm cloth and leave it on for 20-30 minutes.
4. Use this paste once a day to reduce inflammation and improve breathing.

6. **Castor Oil and Thyme Massage Oil**

Ingredients:

- 2 tablespoons castor oil
- 10 drops thyme essential oil

Instructions:

1. Mix castor oil and thyme essential oil in a small bowl.

2. Massage the mixture onto your chest and back, focusing on areas where you feel tightness.
3. Use gentle, circular motions for 5-10 minutes.
4. Apply this massage oil once a day to help open airways and improve respiratory function.

7. **Castor Oil and Lavender Calming Rub**

Ingredients:

- 2 tablespoons castor oil
- 10 drops lavender essential oil

Instructions:

1. Mix castor oil and lavender essential oil in a small bowl.
2. Apply the mixture to your chest, back, and the soles of your feet.
3. Massage gently and cover with warm clothing or a blanket.
4. Use this calming rub before bed to help relax and promote better breathing during sleep.

Note:

- Safety: These recipes are for external use only. Always do a patch test before using any new treatment to ensure you don't have an allergic reaction.
- Consultation: Consult with a healthcare provider before starting any new treatment, especially if you have underlying health conditions or are taking other medications.

Give me 7

1. Castor Oil and Turmeric Paste

Ingredients:

- 2 tablespoons castor oil
- 1 teaspoon ground turmeric
- 1 teaspoon ground ginger (optional)

Instructions:

1. Mix the castor oil, ground turmeric, and ground ginger (if using) in a small bowl to form a thick paste.
2. Apply the paste to the affected joints.
3. Cover with a warm cloth or bandage.
4. Leave it on for 20-30 minutes.
5. Rinse off with warm water.

6. Use this treatment once or twice a day
   to reduce inflammation and pain.

2. **Castor Oil and Epsom Salt Compress**

Ingredients:

- 2 tablespoons castor oil
- 1 tablespoon Epsom salt
- Warm water
- Cloth or bandage

Instructions:

1. Dissolve the Epsom salt in a small
   amount of warm water.
2. Mix the dissolved Epsom salt with the
   castor oil.

3. Soak a cloth or bandage in the mixture.
4. Apply the soaked cloth to the affected joint.
5. Cover with a dry towel and leave it on for 30 minutes.
6. Use this compress once a day to help reduce swelling and relieve pain.

3. Castor Oil and Cayenne Pepper Rub

Ingredients:

- 2 tablespoons castor oil
- 1 teaspoon cayenne pepper powder

Instructions:

1. Mix the castor oil and cayenne pepper powder in a small bowl.

2. Apply a small amount of the mixture to the affected joints, being careful to avoid sensitive skin areas and wash your hands thoroughly afterward.
3. Massage gently for a few minutes.
4. Leave it on for 15-20 minutes.
5. Rinse off with warm water.
6. Use this rub once a day for pain relief.

4. Castor Oil and Essential Oil Massage Blend

Ingredients:

- 2 tablespoons castor oil
- 10 drops lavender essential oil
- 10 drops eucalyptus essential oil

Instructions:

1. Mix the castor oil with lavender and
   eucalyptus essential oils in a small
   bowl.
2. Apply the blend to the affected joints.
3. Massage gently in circular motions for
   5-10 minutes.
4. Use this massage blend twice a day for
   optimal results.

5. Castor Oil and Ginger Compress

Ingredients:

- 2 tablespoons castor oil
- 1 tablespoon grated fresh ginger

Instructions:

1. Warm the castor oil slightly.

2. Add the grated ginger and let it infuse for 10 minutes.
3. Strain out the ginger pieces.
4. Soak a cloth in the warm oil mixture and apply it to the affected joints.
5. Cover with a dry towel and leave it on for 20-30 minutes.
6. Use this compress once a day to relieve inflammation and pain.

6. Castor Oil and Rosemary Salve

Ingredients:

- 2 tablespoons castor oil
- 1 tablespoon beeswax pellets
- 10 drops rosemary essential oil

Instructions:

1. Melt the beeswax pellets in a double boiler.
2. Add the castor oil and mix well until fully combined.
3. Remove from heat and add the rosemary essential oil.
4. Pour the mixture into a small container and let it cool and solidify.
5. Apply a small amount of the salve to the affected joints.
6. Massage gently and use as needed for pain relief.

7. Castor Oil and Arnica Gel

Ingredients:

- 2 tablespoons castor oil
- 1 tablespoon arnica gel

Instructions:

1. Mix the castor oil and arnica gel in a small bowl until well combined.
2. Apply the mixture to the affected joints.
3. Massage gently for a few minutes.
4. Leave it on and allow it to absorb into the skin.
5. Use this treatment twice a day to reduce inflammation and pain.

Note:

- Patch Test: Always perform a patch test before using any new treatment to ensure you don't have an allergic reaction.
- Consultation: Consult with a healthcare provider before starting any new treatment, especially if you have underlying health conditions or are taking other medications.

1. Castor Oil and Epsom Salt Muscle Soak

Ingredients:

- 2 cups Epsom salt
- 2 tablespoons castor oil
- 10 drops lavender essential oil

Instructions:

1. Fill your bathtub with warm water.
2. Add the Epsom salt, castor oil, and lavender essential oil to the water.
3. Stir the water to dissolve the salt and disperse the oils.
4. Soak in the bath for 20-30 minutes.

5. Use this soak once a week to relax muscles and reduce soreness.

2. Castor Oil and Peppermint Massage Oil

Ingredients:

- 2 tablespoons castor oil
- 1 tablespoon coconut oil
- 10 drops peppermint essential oil

Instructions:

1. Mix castor oil and coconut oil in a small bowl.
2. Add peppermint essential oil and stir well.
3. Apply the mixture to sore muscles.

4. Massage gently in circular motions for 5-10 minutes.
5. Use this massage oil as needed to relieve muscle soreness.

3. Castor Oil and Ginger Warm Compress

Ingredients:

- 2 tablespoons castor oil
- 1 tablespoon grated fresh ginger

Instructions:

1. Warm the castor oil slightly.
2. Add the grated ginger and let it infuse for 10 minutes.
3. Strain out the ginger pieces.

4. Soak a cloth in the warm oil mixture and apply it to sore muscles.
5. Cover with a dry towel and leave it on for 20-30 minutes.
6. Use this compress once a day to soothe sore muscles.

4. Castor Oil and Turmeric Muscle Rub

Ingredients:

- 2 tablespoons castor oil
- 1 teaspoon ground turmeric

Instructions:

1. Mix castor oil and ground turmeric in a small bowl to form a paste.

2. Apply the paste to sore muscles.
3. Leave it on for 20-30 minutes.
4. Rinse off with warm water.
5. Use this muscle rub once a day to reduce inflammation and soreness.

5. Castor Oil and Rosemary Muscle Balm

Ingredients:

- 2 tablespoons castor oil
- 1 tablespoon beeswax pellets
- 10 drops rosemary essential oil

Instructions:

1. Melt the beeswax pellets in a double boiler.

2. Add castor oil and mix well until fully combined.
3. Remove from heat and add rosemary essential oil.
4. Pour the mixture into a small container and let it cool and solidify.
5. Apply a small amount of the balm to sore muscles.
6. Massage gently and use as needed for relief.

6. Castor Oil and Arnica Gel Muscle Relief

Ingredients:

- 2 tablespoons castor oil
- 1 tablespoon arnica gel

Instructions:

1. Mix castor oil and arnica gel in a small bowl until well combined.
2. Apply the mixture to sore muscles.
3. Massage gently for a few minutes.
4. Allow it to absorb into the skin.
5. Use this treatment twice a day to reduce muscle soreness.

7. Castor Oil and Eucalyptus Muscle Spray

Ingredients:

- 2 tablespoons castor oil
- 1 cup distilled water
- 10 drops eucalyptus essential oil
- Spray bottle

Instructions:

1. Combine castor oil, distilled water, and eucalyptus essential oil in a spray bottle.
2. Shake well to mix the ingredients.
3. Spray the mixture onto sore muscles.
4. Massage gently until absorbed.
5. Use this spray as needed to relieve muscle soreness.

Note:

- Patch Test: Always perform a patch test before using any new treatment to ensure you don't have an allergic reaction.
- Consultation: Consult with a healthcare provider before starting any new treatment, especially if you have underlying health conditions or are taking other medications.

1. **Castor Oil and Lavender Warm Compress**

Ingredients:

- 2 tablespoons castor oil
- 10 drops lavender essential oil
- Warm water
- Cloth or towel

Instructions:

1. Warm the castor oil slightly.
2. Add the lavender essential oil to the castor oil and mix well.
3. Soak a cloth or towel in warm water and wring out the excess.

4. Apply the oil mixture to your lower abdomen.
5. Place the warm cloth over the area and leave it on for 20-30 minutes.
6. Use this compress once or twice a day during your menstrual cycle to reduce cramps.

2. Castor Oil and Ginger Abdominal Rub

Ingredients:

- 2 tablespoons castor oil
- 1 tablespoon grated fresh ginger

Instructions:

1. Warm the castor oil slightly.

2. Add the grated ginger and let it infuse for 10 minutes.
3. Strain out the ginger pieces.
4. Massage the infused oil onto your lower abdomen in circular motions for 5-10 minutes.
5. Use this rub once or twice a day during your menstrual cycle for relief.

3. Castor Oil and Peppermint Massage Oil

Ingredients:

- 2 tablespoons castor oil
- 1 tablespoon coconut oil
- 10 drops peppermint essential oil

Instructions:

1. Mix the castor oil and coconut oil in a
   small bowl.
2. Add the peppermint essential oil and
   stir well.
3. Massage the mixture onto your lower
   abdomen in gentle, circular motions
   for 5-10 minutes.
4. Use this massage oil as needed to help
   alleviate cramps.

4. Castor Oil and Epsom Salt Bath Soak

Ingredients:

- 2 cups Epsom salt
- 2 tablespoons castor oil
- 10 drops lavender essential oil

Instructions:

1. Fill your bathtub with warm water.
2. Add the Epsom salt, castor oil, and lavender essential oil to the water.
3. Stir the water to dissolve the salt and disperse the oils.
4. Soak in the bath for 20-30 minutes.
5. Use this bath soak once a week or as needed during your menstrual cycle.

5. **Castor Oil and Clary Sage Abdominal Rub**

Ingredients:

- 2 tablespoons castor oil
- 10 drops clary sage essential oil

Instructions:

1. Mix the castor oil and clary sage essential oil in a small bowl.
2. Apply the mixture to your lower abdomen.
3. Massage gently in circular motions for 5-10 minutes.
4. Use this rub once or twice a day during your menstrual cycle to help reduce cramps.

6. **Castor Oil and Chamomile Compress**

Ingredients:

- 2 tablespoons castor oil
- 10 drops chamomile essential oil
- Warm water
- Cloth or towel

Instructions:

1. Warm the castor oil slightly.
2. Add the chamomile essential oil to the castor oil and mix well.
3. Soak a cloth or towel in warm water and wring out the excess.
4. Apply the oil mixture to your lower abdomen.
5. Place the warm cloth over the area and leave it on for 20-30 minutes.
6. Use this compress once or twice a day during your menstrual cycle to ease cramps.

7. **Castor Oil and Cinnamon Warm Rub**

Ingredients:

- 2 tablespoons castor oil
- 1 teaspoon ground cinnamon

Instructions:

1. Warm the castor oil slightly.
2. Add the ground cinnamon and mix well.
3. Apply the mixture to your lower abdomen.
4. Massage gently in circular motions for 5-10 minutes.
5. Cover the area with a warm cloth and leave it on for 20-30 minutes.
6. Use this warm rub once or twice a day during your menstrual cycle to relieve cramps.

Note:

- Patch Test: Always perform a patch test before using any new treatment to ensure you don't have an allergic reaction.

- Consultation: Consult with a healthcare provider before starting any new treatment, especially if you have underlying health conditions or are taking other medications.

Chapter 13: BACK PAIN RECIPES

1. Castor Oil and Epsom Salt Compress

Ingredients:

- 2 tablespoons castor oil
- 1 tablespoon Epsom salt
- Warm water
- Cloth or towel

Instructions:

1. Dissolve the Epsom salt in a small amount of warm water.

2. Mix the dissolved Epsom salt with the castor oil.
3. Soak a cloth or towel in the mixture.
4. Apply the soaked cloth to your back.
5. Cover with a dry towel and leave it on for 20-30 minutes.
6. Use this compress once a day to help reduce back pain and inflammation.

2. Castor Oil and Ginger Compress

Ingredients:

- 2 tablespoons castor oil
- 1 tablespoon grated fresh ginger

Instructions:

1. Warm the castor oil slightly.

2. Add the grated ginger and let it infuse
    for 10 minutes.
3. Strain out the ginger pieces.
4. Soak a cloth in the warm oil mixture
    and apply it to your back.
5. Cover with a dry towel and leave it on
    for 20-30 minutes.
6. Use this compress once a day to
    relieve back pain and muscle tension.

3. Castor Oil and Turmeric Paste

Ingredients:

- 2 tablespoons castor oil
- 1 teaspoon ground turmeric

Instructions:

1. Mix the castor oil and ground turmeric
    in a small bowl to form a thick paste.
2. Apply the paste to the affected area on
    your back.
3. Leave it on for 20-30 minutes.
4. Rinse off with warm water.
5. Use this paste once a day to reduce
    inflammation and pain.

4. Castor Oil and Peppermint Massage Oil

Ingredients:

- 2 tablespoons castor oil
- 1 tablespoon coconut oil
- 10 drops peppermint essential oil

Instructions:

1. Mix the castor oil and coconut oil in a small bowl.
2. Add the peppermint essential oil and stir well.
3. Apply the mixture to your back.
4. Massage gently in circular motions for 5-10 minutes.
5. Use this massage oil as needed to relieve back pain and muscle tension.

5. **Castor Oil and Rosemary Muscle Rub**

Ingredients:

- 2 tablespoons castor oil
- 10 drops rosemary essential oil

Instructions:

1. Mix the castor oil and rosemary essential oil in a small bowl.
2. Apply the mixture to the affected area on your back.
3. Massage gently in circular motions for 5-10 minutes.
4. Use this muscle rub twice a day to reduce back pain and muscle stiffness.

6. Castor Oil and Lavender Compress

Ingredients:

- 2 tablespoons castor oil
- 10 drops lavender essential oil
- Warm water
- Cloth or towel

Instructions:

1. Warm the castor oil slightly.
2. Add the lavender essential oil to the castor oil and mix well.
3. Soak a cloth or towel in warm water and wring out the excess.
4. Apply the oil mixture to your back.
5. Place the warm cloth over the area and leave it on for 20-30 minutes.
6. Use this compress once or twice a day to help reduce back pain and promote relaxation.

7. Castor Oil and Arnica Gel Back Rub

Ingredients:

- 2 tablespoons castor oil
- 1 tablespoon arnica gel

Instructions:

1. Mix the castor oil and arnica gel in a small bowl until well combined.
2. Apply the mixture to the affected area on your back.
3. Massage gently for a few minutes.
4. Allow it to absorb into the skin.
5. Use this treatment twice a day to reduce back pain and inflammation.

Note:

- Patch Test: Always perform a patch test before using any new treatment to ensure you don't have an allergic reaction.
- Consultation: Consult with a healthcare provider before starting any new treatment, especially if you have underlying health conditions or are taking other medications.

1. **Castor Oil and Peppermint Oil Headache Balm**

Ingredients:

- 2 tablespoons castor oil
- 10 drops peppermint essential oil

Instructions:

1. Mix the castor oil and peppermint essential oil in a small bowl.
2. Apply a small amount of the mixture to your temples and forehead.
3. Massage gently in circular motions for a few minutes.
4. Use this balm as needed to relieve headache pain.

2. Castor Oil and Lavender Compress

Ingredients:

- 2 tablespoons castor oil
- 10 drops lavender essential oil
- Warm water
- Cloth or towel

Instructions:

1. Warm the castor oil slightly.
2. Add the lavender essential oil to the castor oil and mix well.
3. Soak a cloth or towel in warm water and wring out the excess.
4. Apply the oil mixture to your forehead and temples.
5. Place the warm cloth over the area and leave it on for 15-20 minutes.

6. Use this compress as needed to help reduce headache pain and promote relaxation.

3. Castor Oil and Eucalyptus Oil Head Massage

Ingredients:

- 2 tablespoons castor oil
- 10 drops eucalyptus essential oil

Instructions:

1. Mix the castor oil and eucalyptus essential oil in a small bowl.
2. Apply the mixture to your temples, forehead, and the back of your neck.
3. Massage gently in circular motions for 5-10 minutes.

4. Use this head massage oil as needed to relieve headache pain and sinus pressure.

4. **Castor Oil and Rosemary Scalp Treatment**

Ingredients:

- 2 tablespoons castor oil
- 10 drops rosemary essential oil

Instructions:

1. Mix the castor oil and rosemary essential oil in a small bowl.
2. Apply the mixture to your scalp, focusing on the areas where you feel tension.

3. Massage gently in circular motions for 5-10 minutes.
4. Leave the oil on for 20-30 minutes, then rinse off with warm water.
5. Use this scalp treatment as needed to relieve tension headaches.

5. **Castor Oil and Chamomile Headache Relief**

Ingredients:

- 2 tablespoons castor oil
- 10 drops chamomile essential oil

Instructions:

1. Mix the castor oil and chamomile essential oil in a small bowl.

2. Apply the mixture to your temples and forehead.
3. Massage gently in circular motions for a few minutes.
4. Use this mixture as needed to help reduce headache pain and promote relaxation.

6. **Castor Oil and Ginger Headache Rub**

Ingredients:

- 2 tablespoons castor oil
- 1 teaspoon grated fresh ginger

Instructions:

1. Warm the castor oil slightly.

2. Add the grated ginger and let it infuse for 10 minutes.
3. Strain out the ginger pieces.
4. Apply the infused oil to your temples and forehead.
5. Massage gently in circular motions for a few minutes.
6. Use this rub as needed to relieve headache pain.

7. **Castor Oil and Clary Sage Aromatherapy**

Ingredients:

- 2 tablespoons castor oil
- 10 drops clary sage essential oil

Instructions:

1. Mix the castor oil and clary sage essential oil in a small bowl.
2. Apply the mixture to your temples, forehead, and the back of your neck.
3. Massage gently in circular motions for 5-10 minutes.
4. Use this aromatherapy treatment as needed to help reduce headache pain and promote relaxation.

Note:

- Patch Test: Always perform a patch test before using any new treatment to ensure you don't have an allergic reaction.
- Consultation: Consult with a healthcare provider before starting any new treatment, especially if you have underlying health conditions or are taking other medications.

1. **Castor Oil Immune Boosting Rub**

Ingredients:

- 2 tablespoons castor oil
- 10 drops tea tree essential oil
- 10 drops eucalyptus essential oil

Instructions:

1. Mix the castor oil, tea tree essential oil, and eucalyptus essential oil in a small bowl.
2. Apply the mixture to your chest and neck.
3. Massage gently in circular motions for 5-10 minutes.

4. Use this rub once a day to help support your immune system.

2. Castor Oil and Garlic Immune Boosting Pack

Ingredients:

- 2 tablespoons castor oil
- 2 cloves garlic, minced
- Cloth or bandage

Instructions:

1. Warm the castor oil slightly.
2. Add the minced garlic and let it infuse for 15 minutes.
3. Strain out the garlic pieces.

4. Soak a cloth or bandage in the infused oil.
5. Apply the cloth to your abdomen and leave it on for 20-30 minutes.
6. Use this pack once a day to help support immune function.

3. **Castor Oil and Ginger Immune Tonic**

Ingredients:

- 1 teaspoon castor oil
- 1 teaspoon grated fresh ginger
- 1 cup hot water
- 1 teaspoon honey (optional)

Instructions:

1. Add the grated ginger to a cup of hot water and let it steep for 5-10 minutes.
2. Strain the ginger tea into a cup.
3. Add the castor oil and honey (if using) to the ginger tea.
4. Stir well and drink this tonic once a day to help support your immune system.

4. Castor Oil and Lemon Immune Boosting Drink

Ingredients:

- 1 teaspoon castor oil
- Juice of 1 lemon
- 1 cup warm water
- 1 teaspoon honey (optional)

Instructions:

1. Mix the lemon juice, castor oil, and honey (if using) in a cup of warm water.
2. Stir well until fully combined.
3. Drink this mixture once a day to help support your immune system.

5. Castor Oil and Turmeric Immune Boosting Paste

Ingredients:

- 2 tablespoons castor oil
- 1 teaspoon ground turmeric
- 1 teaspoon honey

Instructions:

1. Mix the castor oil, ground turmeric, and honey in a small bowl to form a paste.
2. Take 1 teaspoon of the paste daily, either on its own or mixed into a warm beverage.
3. Use this paste once a day to help support your immune system.

6. **Castor Oil and Oregano Immune Support Capsules**

Ingredients:

- 1 teaspoon castor oil
- 5 drops oregano essential oil
- Empty gelatin capsules

Instructions:

1. Mix the castor oil and oregano essential oil in a small bowl.
2. Use a dropper to fill empty gelatin capsules with the mixture.
3. Take one capsule daily to help support your immune system.

7. **Castor Oil Immune Support Massage Oil**

Ingredients:

- 2 tablespoons castor oil
- 10 drops rosemary essential oil
- 10 drops lavender essential oil

Instructions:

1. Mix the castor oil, rosemary essential oil, and lavender essential oil in a small bowl.
2. Apply the mixture to your back, chest, and neck.
3. Massage gently in circular motions for 5-10 minutes.
4. Use this massage oil once a day to help support your immune system.

Note:

- Patch Test: Always perform a patch test before using any new topical treatment to ensure you don't have an allergic reaction.
- Consultation: Consult with a healthcare provider before starting any new treatment, especially if you have underlying health conditions, are pregnant or nursing, or are taking other medications.

1. **Castor Oil Hair Growth Serum**

Ingredients:

- 2 tablespoons castor oil
- 1 tablespoon coconut oil
- 5 drops rosemary essential oil
- 5 drops peppermint essential oil

Instructions:

1. Mix all ingredients in a small bowl until well combined.
2. Apply the serum to your scalp and massage gently for 5-10 minutes.
3. Leave the serum on for at least 30 minutes or overnight.
4. Wash your hair with shampoo and conditioner as usual.

5. Use this serum 2-3 times per week for promoting hair growth.

2. Castor Oil Deep Conditioning Mask

Ingredients:

- 2 tablespoons castor oil
- 1 tablespoon honey
- 1 ripe avocado

Instructions:

1. Mash the avocado in a bowl until smooth.
2. Add castor oil and honey to the mashed avocado and mix well.
3. Apply the mixture to damp hair, focusing on the ends and damaged areas.

4. Leave the mask on for 30-60 minutes.
5. Rinse thoroughly with warm water and shampoo.
6. Use this deep conditioning mask once a week for soft and nourished hair.

3. **Castor Oil and Aloe Vera Scalp Treatment**

Ingredients:

- 2 tablespoons castor oil
- 2 tablespoons aloe vera gel

Instructions:

1. Mix castor oil and aloe vera gel in a bowl until well combined.

2. Apply the mixture directly to your scalp and massage gently for 5-10 minutes.
3. Leave the treatment on for 30 minutes to an hour.
4. Rinse thoroughly with lukewarm water and shampoo.
5. Use this scalp treatment 1-2 times per week to soothe the scalp and promote healthy hair growth.

4. Castor Oil and Egg Protein Hair Mask

Ingredients:

- 2 tablespoons castor oil
- 1 egg
- 1 tablespoon yogurt

Instructions:

1. Beat the egg in a bowl until frothy.
2. Add castor oil and yogurt to the beaten egg and mix well.
3. Apply the mixture to damp hair, focusing on the roots and ends.
4. Leave the mask on for 30-45 minutes.
5. Rinse thoroughly with cool water and shampoo.
6. Use this protein-rich hair mask once a week to strengthen and nourish your hair.

5. Castor Oil and Jojoba Oil Hair Serum

Ingredients:

- 2 tablespoons castor oil
- 1 tablespoon jojoba oil
- 5 drops lavender essential oil

Instructions:

1. Mix castor oil, jojoba oil, and lavender essential oil in a small bottle.
2. Apply a few drops of the serum to your fingertips and massage into the scalp.
3. Brush the serum through your hair, focusing on the ends.
4. Leave the serum in overnight or wash it out after a few hours.
5. Use this hair serum 2-3 times per week for added moisture and shine.

6. Castor Oil and Coconut Milk Hair Mask

Ingredients:

- 2 tablespoons castor oil
- 1/4 cup coconut milk

- 1 tablespoon honey

Instructions:

1. Mix castor oil, coconut milk, and honey in a bowl until well combined.
2. Apply the mixture to damp hair, focusing on the scalp and roots.
3. Cover your hair with a shower cap and leave the mask on for 30-60 minutes.
4. Rinse thoroughly with warm water and shampoo.
5. Use this nourishing hair mask once a week for soft, manageable hair.

7. Castor Oil and Green Tea Rinse

Ingredients:

- 2 tablespoons castor oil

- 1 cup brewed green tea, cooled

Instructions:

1. Mix castor oil and cooled green tea in a bowl.
2. After shampooing and conditioning your hair, pour the mixture over your scalp and hair.
3. Massage gently for a few minutes to distribute evenly.
4. Leave the rinse on for 5-10 minutes.
5. Rinse thoroughly with cool water.
6. Use this green tea rinse once or twice a week to stimulate hair growth and improve scalp health.

Chapter 17: NAILS CARE RECIPES

1. Castor Oil Nail Strengthener

Ingredients:

- 1 tablespoon castor oil
- 1 tablespoon argan oil
- 5 drops lemon essential oil

Instructions:

1. Mix all ingredients in a small bowl.
2. Massage the mixture onto your nails and cuticles.
3. Leave it on for at least 15 minutes or overnight.
4. Rinse off or wipe away any excess oil.
5. Use this nail strengthener daily or as needed to strengthen and nourish your nails.

2. Castor Oil and Vitamin E Cuticle Oil

Ingredients:

- 1 tablespoon castor oil
- 1 teaspoon vitamin E oil
- 3 drops lavender essential oil (optional)

Instructions:

1. Mix castor oil, vitamin E oil, and lavender essential oil (if using) in a small bowl.
2. Apply a small amount of the mixture to each nail and massage into the cuticles.
3. Leave it on for 10-15 minutes.
4. Wipe away any excess oil.
5. Use this cuticle oil daily to moisturize and strengthen your nails.

3. Castor Oil and Coconut Oil Nail Soak

Ingredients:

- 1 tablespoon castor oil
- 1 tablespoon coconut oil
- Warm water

Instructions:

1. Mix castor oil and coconut oil in a small bowl.
2. Soak your nails in warm water for 5-10 minutes to soften them.
3. Pat dry and apply the oil mixture to your nails and cuticles.
4. Massage gently for a few minutes.
5. Leave it on for 15-20 minutes.
6. Rinse off or wipe away any excess oil.
7. Use this nail soak once a week to hydrate and nourish your nails.

4. **Castor Oil and Olive Oil Nail Mask**

Ingredients:

- 1 tablespoon castor oil
- 1 tablespoon olive oil
- 1 teaspoon honey

Instructions:

1. Mix castor oil, olive oil, and honey in a small bowl.
2. Apply the mixture to your nails and cuticles.
3. Leave it on for 15-20 minutes.
4. Rinse off or wipe away any excess oil.
5. Use this nail mask once a week to moisturize and strengthen your nails.

5. **Castor Oil and Shea Butter Nail Balm**

Ingredients:

- 1 tablespoon castor oil
- 1 tablespoon shea butter
- 5 drops rosemary essential oil

Instructions:

1. Melt the shea butter in a double boiler.
2. Once melted, remove from heat and stir in castor oil and rosemary essential oil.
3. Allow the mixture to cool slightly.
4. Apply a small amount to your nails and cuticles.
5. Massage gently until absorbed.

6. Use this nail balm daily to moisturize and protect your nails.

6. **Castor Oil and Tea Tree Oil Nail Treatment**

Ingredients:

- 1 tablespoon castor oil
- 3 drops tea tree essential oil

Instructions:

1. Mix castor oil and tea tree essential oil in a small bowl.
2. Apply a small amount of the mixture to each nail and massage into the cuticles.
3. Leave it on for 10-15 minutes.

4. Wipe away any excess oil.
5. Use this nail treatment daily to strengthen and protect your nails.

7. **Castor Oil and Lemon Juice Nail Whitener**

Ingredients:

- 1 tablespoon castor oil
- Juice of half a lemon

Instructions:

1. Mix castor oil and lemon juice in a small bowl.
2. Soak your nails in the mixture for 5-10 minutes.

3. Rinse off with warm water and pat dry.
4. Use this nail whitening treatment once a week to brighten and strengthen your nails.

Chapter 18:SKIN CARE RECIPES

1. Castor Oil Cleansing Oil

Ingredients:

- 2 tablespoons castor oil
- 1 tablespoon olive oil or jojoba oil
- 5 drops lavender essential oil (optional)

Instructions:

1. Mix all ingredients in a small bottle.

2. Apply a small amount of the oil mixture to your dry skin.

3. Massage gently in circular motions for 1-2 minutes.

4. Wet a washcloth with warm water and wring out excess.

5. Use the warm washcloth to gently wipe away the oil.

6. Rinse your face with lukewarm water and pat dry.

7. Use this cleansing oil nightly to remove makeup and impurities without stripping your skin.

2. Castor Oil and Honey Face Mask

Ingredients:

- 1 tablespoon castor oil
- 1 tablespoon raw honey

Instructions:

1. Mix castor oil and honey in a small bowl until well combined.
2. Apply the mixture to your clean face, avoiding the eye area.
3. Leave the mask on for 15-20 minutes.
4. Rinse off with lukewarm water and pat dry.
5. Use this face mask once a week to hydrate, soothe, and clarify your skin.

3. Castor Oil and Sugar Scrub

Ingredients:

- 2 tablespoons castor oil
- 1 tablespoon brown sugar

Instructions:

1. Mix castor oil and brown sugar in a small bowl until well combined.
2. Gently massage the scrub onto damp skin in circular motions for 1-2 minutes.
3. Rinse off with warm water and pat dry.
4. Follow up with a moisturizer.
5. Use this scrub 2-3 times a week to exfoliate and smooth your skin.

4. Castor Oil and Aloe Vera Gel Moisturizer

Ingredients:

- 2 tablespoons castor oil
- 1 tablespoon aloe vera gel

Instructions:

1. Mix castor oil and aloe vera gel in a small bowl until well combined.
2. Apply the mixture to your clean, dry skin.
3. Massage gently until absorbed.
4. Use this moisturizer daily to hydrate and soothe your skin, especially after sun exposure.

5. Castor Oil and Green Tea Toner

Ingredients:

- 2 tablespoons castor oil
- 1/4 cup brewed green tea, cooled

Instructions:

1. Mix castor oil and cooled green tea in a small bottle.

2. After cleansing your face, apply a small amount of the mixture to a cotton pad.
3. Swipe the toner over your face and neck, avoiding the eye area.
4. Allow it to air dry.
5. Follow up with your regular skincare routine.
6. Use this toner daily to tighten pores and balance your skin's pH.

6. **Castor Oil and Oatmeal Bath Soak**

Ingredients:

- 2 tablespoons castor oil
- 1/2 cup oats (ground into a fine powder)
- 1/4 cup milk or almond milk

Instructions:

1. Mix castor oil, oatmeal powder, and milk in a bathtub filled with warm water.
2. Stir well to dissolve the ingredients.
3. Soak in the bath for 15-20 minutes.
4. Rinse off with lukewarm water and pat dry.
5. Use this bath soak once a week to soothe and moisturize dry, irritated skin.

7. Castor Oil and Chamomile Eye Cream

Ingredients:

- 1 tablespoon castor oil
- 1 tablespoon shea butter
- 5 drops chamomile essential oil

Instructions:

1. Melt the shea butter in a double boiler.
2. Once melted, remove from heat and stir in castor oil and chamomile essential oil.
3. Allow the mixture to cool and solidify.
4. Apply a small amount of the eye cream around your eyes, avoiding direct contact with the eyes.
5. Gently pat until absorbed.
6. Use this eye cream nightly to moisturize and reduce puffiness around the eyes.

Chapter 19: EYES RECIPES

1. Castor Oil Eye Serum for Moisturizing

Ingredients:

- 1 tablespoon castor oil
- 1 teaspoon sweet almond oil
- 3 drops vitamin E oil

Instructions:

1. Mix all the oils in a small dropper bottle.
2. Shake well to ensure they are thoroughly combined.
3. Apply a drop or two of the serum around the eyes.
4. Gently massage in circular motions until absorbed.
5. Use daily, preferably before bedtime, to keep the delicate skin around the eyes moisturized.

2. Castor Oil and Cucumber Eye Mask for Puffiness

Ingredients:

- 1 tablespoon castor oil

- 1/4 cucumber (peeled and grated)

Instructions:

1. Mix the grated cucumber with castor oil in a small bowl.
2. Refrigerate the mixture for about 30 minutes.
3. Take a small amount and apply it to the area around your eyes.
4. Leave on for 10-15 minutes.
5. Rinse off with cool water and pat dry.
6. Use this mask 2-3 times a week to reduce puffiness and refresh tired eyes.

3. **Castor Oil and Rosewater Soothing Eye Compress**

Ingredients:

- 1 tablespoon castor oil
- 2 tablespoons rosewater
- Cotton pads or balls

Instructions:

1. Mix castor oil and rosewater in a small bowl.
2. Soak cotton pads or balls in the mixture.
3. Lie down and place the soaked pads over closed eyes.
4. Relax for 10-15 minutes.
5. Remove pads and gently massage any excess oil into the skin.
6. Use this compress as needed to soothe and rejuvenate tired eyes.

4. Castor Oil and Aloe Vera Gel Eye Gel for Dark Circles

Ingredients:

- 1 tablespoon castor oil
- 1 tablespoon aloe vera gel

Instructions:

1. Mix castor oil and aloe vera gel in a small bowl.
2. Apply a small amount of the mixture under the eyes.
3. Gently massage in circular motions until absorbed.
4. Leave it on overnight.
5. Rinse off with lukewarm water in the morning.
6. Use this gel nightly to reduce dark circles and hydrate the under-eye area.

5. Castor Oil and Green Tea Eye Toner

Ingredients:

- 1 tablespoon castor oil
- 1/4 cup brewed green tea, cooled

Instructions:

1. Mix castor oil and cooled green tea in a small bottle.
2. After cleansing your face, apply a small amount of the mixture to a cotton pad.
3. Swipe the toner over closed eyes.
4. Allow it to air dry.
5. Follow up with your regular skincare routine.
6. Use this toner daily to reduce puffiness and soothe the eye area.

6. **Castor Oil and Potato Eye Mask for Brightening**

Ingredients:

- 1 tablespoon castor oil
- 1/4 potato (peeled and grated)

Instructions:

1. Mix the grated potato with castor oil in a small bowl.
2. Apply the mixture around the eyes.
3. Leave on for 15-20 minutes.
4. Rinse off with cool water and pat dry.
5. Use this mask 2-3 times a week to brighten and lighten dark circles.

7. **Castor Oil and Chamomile Eye Cream for Wrinkles**

Ingredients:

- 1 tablespoon castor oil
- 1 tablespoon shea butter
- 5 drops chamomile essential oil

Instructions:

1. Melt the shea butter in a double boiler.
2. Once melted, remove from heat and stir in castor oil and chamomile essential oil.
3. Allow the mixture to cool and solidify.
4. Apply a small amount of the eye cream around your eyes, avoiding direct contact with the eyes.
5. Gently pat until absorbed.

6. Use this eye cream nightly to moisturize and reduce the appearance of fine lines and wrinkles.

Chapter 20:BODY CARE RECIPES

1. Castor Oil Body Moisturizer

Ingredients:

- 1/4 cup castor oil
- 1/4 cup coconut oil
- 1/4 cup shea butter
- 10 drops lavender essential oil (optional)

Instructions:

1. In a double boiler, melt the coconut oil and shea butter until fully liquid.

2. Remove from heat and stir in the castor oil and lavender essential oil (if using).
3. Let the mixture cool until slightly thickened.
4. Transfer to a clean jar or container.
5. Apply to damp skin after showering, focusing on dry areas like elbows and knees.
6. Use daily for soft, hydrated skin.

2. Castor Oil Body Scrub

Ingredients:

- 1/2 cup brown sugar
- 1/4 cup castor oil
- 1/4 cup honey
- 1 teaspoon vanilla extract (optional)

Instructions:

1. Mix all ingredients in a bowl until well combined.
2. Apply the scrub to damp skin in the shower, using gentle circular motions.
3. Focus on rough areas like elbows, knees, and feet.
4. Rinse off with warm water.
5. Pat skin dry and follow up with a moisturizer.
6. Use 2-3 times a week for smooth, exfoliated skin.

3. **Castor Oil Massage Oil for Relaxation**

Ingredients:

- 1/4 cup castor oil
- 1/4 cup sweet almond oil
- 10 drops lavender essential oil
- 5 drops peppermint essential oil

Instructions:

1. Mix all ingredients in a small bottle or jar.
2. Shake well to blend the oils.
3. Warm a small amount of oil between your palms.
4. Massage into the skin using long, gentle strokes.
5. Focus on areas of tension or soreness.
6. Use as needed for a relaxing massage experience.

4. Castor Oil Foot Balm

Ingredients:

- 1/4 cup castor oil
- 2 tablespoons beeswax pellets
- 2 tablespoons cocoa butter
- 10 drops tea tree essential oil

- 5 drops peppermint essential oil

Instructions:

1. In a double boiler, melt the beeswax and cocoa butter until fully liquid.
2. Remove from heat and stir in the castor oil and essential oils.
3. Pour the mixture into a clean container.
4. Allow to cool and solidify.
5. Massage into clean, dry feet, focusing on rough areas.
6. Put on socks and leave overnight for maximum hydration.
7. Use regularly to keep feet soft and smooth.

5. Castor Oil Body Butter

Ingredients:

- 1/2 cup shea butter
- 1/4 cup castor oil
- 1/4 cup coconut oil
- 10 drops vanilla essential oil (optional)

Instructions:

1. In a double boiler, melt the shea butter and coconut oil until fully liquid.
2. Remove from heat and stir in the castor oil and vanilla essential oil (if using).
3. Let the mixture cool slightly, then transfer to a mixing bowl.
4. Whip the mixture using a hand mixer until light and fluffy.
5. Transfer to a clean jar or container.
6. Apply to skin as needed for deep hydration.

6. **Castor Oil Body Lotion Bar**

Ingredients:

- 1/4 cup castor oil
- 1/4 cup cocoa butter
- 1/4 cup beeswax pellets
- 10 drops lavender essential oil

Instructions:

1. In a double boiler, melt the cocoa butter and beeswax pellets until fully liquid.
2. Remove from heat and stir in the castor oil and lavender essential oil.
3. Pour the mixture into molds or a silicone ice cube tray.
4. Let it cool and harden at room temperature or in the refrigerator.

5. Once solid, remove from molds and store in a cool, dry place.
6. To use, rub the lotion bar between your hands to warm it up, then massage onto skin for moisturization.

7. Castor Oil Cuticle Cream

Ingredients:

- 2 tablespoons castor oil
- 1 tablespoon shea butter
- 1 tablespoon coconut oil
- 5 drops lemon essential oil

Instructions:

1. In a double boiler, melt the shea butter and coconut oil until fully liquid.

2. Remove from heat and stir in the castor oil and lemon essential oil.
3. Pour the mixture into a small jar or container.
4. Allow it to cool and solidify.
5. Apply a small amount to your cuticles and massage in gently.
6. Use daily to moisturize and condition your cuticles.

Chapter 21:MENTAL AND EMOTIONAL WELL-BEING RECIPES

1. Castor Oil Relaxation Bath Blend

Ingredients:

- 1/4 cup castor oil
- 1/2 cup Epsom salt
- 5 drops lavender essential oil
- 3 drops chamomile essential oil

Instructions:

1. Fill your bathtub with warm water.
2. Add the castor oil and Epsom salt to the water.
3. Stir the mixture until the Epsom salt dissolves.
4. Add the lavender and chamomile essential oils.
5. Soak in the bath for 15-20 minutes, allowing the calming scents and properties of castor oil to relax your mind and body.
6. Take slow, deep breaths and focus on releasing tension with each exhale.

2. Castor Oil Aromatherapy Diffuser Blend

Ingredients:

- 5 drops castor oil
- 3 drops bergamot essential oil
- 2 drops ylang-ylang essential oil

Instructions:

1. Fill your aromatherapy diffuser with water.
2. Add the castor oil, bergamot essential oil, and ylang-ylang essential oil to the water.
3. Turn on the diffuser and let the calming aroma fill the room.
4. Sit quietly and breathe deeply, allowing the scent to promote relaxation and ease stress.
5. Practice mindfulness or meditation while enjoying the aromatherapy experience.

3. Castor Oil Stress-Relief Massage Oil

Ingredients:

- 2 tablespoons castor oil
- 1 tablespoon sweet almond oil
- 5 drops rosemary essential oil
- 3 drops peppermint essential oil

Instructions:

1. Mix all ingredients in a small bottle or jar.
2. Shake well to blend the oils.
3. Warm a small amount of the oil between your palms.
4. Massage into your neck, shoulders, and any other areas of tension.
5. Take slow, deep breaths as you massage, allowing the soothing properties of castor oil and essential oils to ease stress and promote relaxation.

4. **Castor Oil Calming Pillow Spray**

Ingredients:

- 1 tablespoon castor oil
- 2 tablespoons witch hazel
- 5 drops lavender essential oil
- 3 drops cedarwood essential oil

Instructions:

1. Mix castor oil, witch hazel, and essential oils in a small spray bottle.
2. Shake well to combine the ingredients.
3. Spritz the calming spray lightly onto your pillow before bedtime.
4. Lie down and take slow, deep breaths, inhaling the soothing aroma of lavender and cedarwood.

5. Allow yourself to relax fully, releasing any tension or worries as you drift off to sleep.

5. Castor Oil Self-Care Roll-On Blend

Ingredients:

- 1 tablespoon castor oil
- 3 drops geranium essential oil
- 2 drops frankincense essential oil
- 2 drops bergamot essential oil

Instructions:

1. Mix castor oil and essential oils in a small roll-on bottle.
2. Roll the blend onto pulse points such as wrists, temples, and behind the ears.

3. Take a moment to inhale the uplifting scents and set an intention for self-care and emotional well-being.
4. Throughout the day, return to these pulse points, taking deep breaths and reminding yourself of your intention to prioritize your mental and emotional health.

CONCLUSION

In closing, "The Castor Oil Bible" offers a comprehensive guide to unlocking the myriad benefits of this remarkable natural remedy. With its rich historical background, detailed extraction methods, and extensive array of recipes for health, beauty, and well-being, this book serves as a trusted companion on your journey to holistic living.

Through the pages of "The Castor Oil Bible," readers are empowered to harness the healing power of castor oil in every aspect of their lives, from physical wellness to mental and emotional balance. Whether you're seeking relief from ailments, enhancing your beauty regimen, or simply looking to embrace a more natural lifestyle, this book provides the knowledge and inspiration to do so with confidence.

With its accessible language, practical tips, and enticing recipes, "The Castor Oil Bible" invites readers to embark on a transformative journey towards vibrant health and radiant beauty. It's more than just a book—it's a roadmap to wellness, a treasure trove of wisdom, and a testament to the remarkable potential of nature's gifts.

Discover the endless possibilities of castor oil and unlock a world of health, beauty, and vitality. Embrace the wisdom of "The Castor Oil Bible" and embark on a journey to holistic well-being today.

THE END